DEFEATING ASTHMA WITH EXPERT GUIDANCE

Ultimate Solution Handbook For Patients,
Guardians Or Family To Understand,
Manage, Treat, Prevent, Reverse Symptoms
And Live Well

DR. POTTER WHITLEY

Copyright © 2023 by Dr. Potter Whitley

DISCLAIMER:

This book's contents are meant to be used solely for informative purposes. The information should not be used as a replacement for expert medical advice, diagnosis, or care.

The information contained in this book is accurate and reliable, having been verified by the author to the best of his ability. Nevertheless, the author disclaims all express and implied representations and warranties regarding the availability, correctness, appropriateness, completeness, and reliability of the material provided here. You bear full responsibility for any reliance you may have on such material.

For informational purposes, this book may make reference to or mention of certain people, things, websites, organizations, or other names. The author has no connection to, endorsement from, or recommendation for these organizations. The author's approval or validation is not implied by the inclusion of these references.

Any direct, indirect, incidental, special, or consequential damages resulting from using or not being able to use the material in this book are not covered by the author's liability policy. For medical advice and counsel particular to their circumstances, readers are advised to check with experienced healthcare specialists.

The content, materials, and information in this book are subject to change at any time without prior notice, at the author's discretion. The text may contain errors or omissions for which the author is not responsible.

By reading this book, you understand and accept the conditions of this disclaimer.

THE REASON BEHIND THIS BOOK

For anyone struggling with asthma, "Defeating ASTHMA With Expert Guidance" is a priceless resource that provides a thorough understanding of the illness and a management road map. Asthma has a widespread impact on daily life, and the opening part lays out the background by highlighting the importance of expert help in navigating its intricacies. Readers are brought through the complexities of asthma as the story progresses, from its description and types to an examination of its causes and triggers, all of which are presented understandably and straightforwardly.

The book's emphasis on the value of a precise diagnosis and comprehensive evaluation is one of its strongest points; it gives readers the tools they need to identify symptoms, be tested for diseases, and comprehend the severity and categorization of their conditions. By discussing the collaborative nature of managing asthma, promoting a solid patient-doctor relationship, and outlining the responsibilities of specialists within the larger healthcare team, the work adopts a holistic approach.

Examining asthma medication options is especially instructive, as it offers a summary of what's available, tips for using nebulizers and inhalers, and insights into how to manage prescription regimens. The book explores environmental and lifestyle issues in addition to medical therapies, stressing the importance of leading a healthy lifestyle and providing helpful tips for making a home asthma-friendly.

The book stands out for its thorough treatment of nutrition, which explains the complex relationship between food and asthma control. It defies accepted knowledge by investigating items that might lessen symptoms and providing preventative dietary strategies. The conversation moves on to physical activity, emphasizing the advantages of exercise for those with asthma, helping readers choose appropriate activities, and describing the safety precautions that must be taken.

As the story goes on, the book looks into complementary and alternative medicines, recognizing how the field of asthma care is changing. It recognizes the unique factors that need to be taken into account when managing asthma in various age groups, with a focus on children, adolescents, and seniors. The work's conclusion takes a forward-looking approach, examining new developments in research, technology, and treatment options that show promise and offer an overview of how asthma care is developing.

"Defeating ASTHMA With Expert Guidance" essentially goes beyond the accepted bounds of medical knowledge. Its lively and sophisticated style, along with a thorough examination of asthma from multiple perspectives, make it an invaluable resource for anybody looking for more than simply information—rather, a how-to manual for taking charge of their respiratory well-being.

TABLE OF CONTENT

CHAPTER ONE

<u>OVERVIEW</u>
<u>An Overview of Allergies</u>

Millions of individuals worldwide suffer from asthma, a chronic respiratory disease that is characterized by airway constriction and inflammation. Recurrent episodes of wheezing, dyspnea, tightness in the chest, and coughing may result from this condition. The primary cause of asthma is the airways' responsiveness to several stimuli, including exercise, irritants, and allergens. The muscles around the airways contract and the lining of the air passageways expands during an asthma episode, which reduces airflow. This may set off a chain reaction of symptoms that have a major negative influence on people's psychological and emotional health in addition to their physical health.

Managing a daily schedule that is frequently impacted by the unpredictable nature of symptoms is part of having asthma. Since abrupt exacerbations can interrupt times of relative normalcy for those who have asthma, it's critical to successfully manage the condition. The difficulties go beyond the physical symptoms to include the lifestyle modifications needed to reduce triggers and preserve lung function at its best. To manage and lessen the effects of this chronic illness, people with asthma and their families must have a thorough understanding of the nature of the disease, its triggers, and the mechanisms underlying its symptoms.

How Asthma Affects Everyday Life:

The impact of asthma goes well beyond the body and has a big impact on the everyday lives of people who have been diagnosed with it. Asthma symptoms can be erratic, which can interfere with daily activities and make participation in a variety of activities more difficult. For those who have asthma, even seemingly easy things like walking in the cold or climbing stairs can become extremely difficult. Moreover, social interactions and outdoor activities may be restricted due to the ongoing need to be aware of potential triggers, such as allergies or environmental pollution.

It's important to recognize the psychological toll that having asthma takes in addition to its physical limitations. Anxiety and a lower quality of life might be brought on by the fear of unexpected asthma episodes, the frustration of being unable to participate in particular activities, and the possible stigma attached to the condition. The effects of asthma extend beyond the person with the diagnosis to include family members and caregivers, who must adjust to the difficulties the illness presents. An all-encompassing strategy for managing asthma must acknowledge and treat its complex effects.

The Value of Professional Advice in the Management of Asthma

In the complex world of asthma control, professional advice plays a critical role. Even while people may get a general awareness of their disease, individualized and successful management depends on the knowledge of healthcare professionals. Since no two people with asthma are the same, treating the illness appropriately necessitates taking into account each person's particular triggers, symptoms, and lifestyle choices.

Professionals in the medical field, such as pulmonologists, allergists, and asthma educators, are essential in equipping people with the information and abilities required to manage their asthma.

They offer thorough evaluations, inform patients about their condition, and create individualized action plans that enable people to manage their asthma. Expert advice includes lifestyle modifications, trigger detection, and preventative steps to avoid exacerbations in addition to medicinal therapies.

In summary, an all-encompassing strategy that goes beyond simple symptom management is required to fight asthma. A comprehensive asthma treatment plan must recognize the subtleties of the condition, acknowledge its influence on day-to-day living, and seek professional advice.

By working together, patients, medical professionals, and support systems may improve the lives of those who are impacted by asthma and create a future in which the difficulties brought on by this long-term illness are successfully addressed.

CHAPTER TWO

KNOWING ABOUT ASTHMA
Asthma Definition and Types:

Chronic asthma is a respiratory disease that causes inflammation of the airways, which frequently results in wheezing fits, dyspnea, tightness in the chest, and coughing fits. The illness results from a complicated interaction between environmental and hereditary variables. People who have asthma have hypersensitive airways that react strongly to a variety of stimuli, frequently narrowing and obstructing them.

Asthma comes in various forms, each with distinct features. The most prevalent type of asthma, allergic asthma, is brought on by exposure to allergens such as dust mites, pollen, or pet dander. Conversely, non-allergic asthma can be brought on by things like exertion, stress, or respiratory infections. While nocturnal asthma typically gets worse at night, occupational asthma is linked to certain exposures at work. Comprehending the particular form of asthma is essential to customizing efficacious treatment approaches.

Reasons and Initiators:

The etiology of asthma is complex and involves both environmental and genetic variables. People who have a family history of asthma or other allergies are more vulnerable. The onset or worsening of asthma symptoms might be caused by exposure to specific environmental factors. Dust mites, pet dander, mold spores, and pollen are examples of common allergies. Significant contributions also come from environmental contaminants including air pollution and tobacco smoke.

In addition to allergens and pollution, respiratory infections—particularly in the early stages of childhood—can raise the risk of developing asthma. Asthma at work can also result from occupational exposure to allergens like dust or chemical fumes. In certain people, emotional issues such as stress and anxiety can exacerbate asthma symptoms.

Identifying and staying away from triggers is essential for asthma management. People who have asthma should create a customized asthma action plan with medical specialists. This plan should include techniques for avoiding triggers and early warning indicators of an imminent exacerbation.

The Effects of Asthma on the Respiratory System:

The respiratory system, and more especially the bronchial tubes that transport air to and from the lungs, is the primary target of asthma's effects. Asthma sufferers experience inflammation of the airways, which increases mucus production and causes bronchial wall enlargement. The muscles that surround the airways may also tighten, making the passageways even smaller.

These modifications cause airflow to be obstructed, making breathing difficult for some people. This airflow restriction manifests as the usual asthma symptoms: wheezing, shortness of breath, chest tightness, and coughing. The degree of symptoms during an asthma attack can vary, from mild to potentially fatal, underscoring the need for timely and effective therapy.

Uncontrolled asthma may have long-term effects, such as airway remodeling, a condition in which the airways' structural makeup alterations with time and results in a persistent restriction of airflow. This emphasizes how important it is to manage asthma well and promptly to lessen its negative effects on the respiratory system and general quality of life.

CHAPTER THREE

DIAGNOSIS AND EVALUATION
Identifying Symptoms of Asthma

Identifying the symptoms of asthma is an essential first step toward treating and managing this long-term respiratory disease. The hallmark of asthma is inflammation of the airways, which results in symptoms including coughing, chest tightness, wheezing, and shortness of breath. Since the frequency and severity of these symptoms might vary, early detection is crucial for prompt action.

The characteristic sound of asthma is wheezing, which is a high-pitched whistling sound made during breathing. It usually happens as you exhale and is caused by your airways becoming narrower. Another typical symptom is shortness of breath, which is caused by restricted airflow from the inflamed airways, making it difficult for people to breathe deeply. Another sign of asthma is chest tightness, which is frequently described as a sense of pressure or constriction in the chest.

Coughing is another symptom that has to be addressed, particularly if it occurs at night or in response to a particular trigger. Coughs caused by asthma are oftentimes chronic and in certain instances the only symptom. Acknowledging these symptoms is essential for both patients and medical professionals, as early diagnosis and treatment can greatly enhance the quality of life for asthma sufferers.

Furthermore, it's critical to comprehend how symptoms can vary. Asthma exacerbations are episodes when symptoms of the disease worsen due to certain circumstances or triggers. Effective therapy of asthma necessitates the identification of these triggers, which might vary from allergies to respiratory infections. Using a peak flow meter or symptom journal to regularly record symptoms can help track changes and give medical practitioners useful information.

To put it briefly, identifying the symptoms of asthma entails having a thorough awareness of all of its many expressions, which range from chest tightness and chronic coughing to wheezing and shortness of breath. Early detection lessens the effect of asthma on day-to-day functioning and averts serious exacerbations by enabling patients and medical professionals to take prompt action.

Diagnostic Procedures and Tests

Precise diagnosis of asthma necessitates a blend of clinical assessment and particular diagnostic techniques and processes. Asthma's existence and severity can be objectively confirmed by particular tests, even though the clinical history and physical examination are still very important. These diagnostic tools help medical practitioners create an asthma treatment plan that works for patients.

Spirometry, a lung function test that gauges the volume and rate of air exhaled from the lungs, is one of the main diagnostic procedures. Asthma is characterized by airflow limitation, which is evaluated with the aid of spirometry. Furthermore, bronchoprovocation testing can be performed to cause airway constriction and validate the diagnosis, especially in cases when spirometry data are unclear.

Asthma triggers can worsen symptoms, thus allergy testing is a crucial part of the diagnosing process. Certain allergens that may be aggravating asthma symptoms can be found using skin or blood testing. Determining and controlling these triggers is essential for long-term asthma management that works.

Imaging tests, including computed tomography (CT) scans or chest X-rays, may be used in some situations to assess the degree of airway inflammation and rule out other respiratory disorders. These imaging techniques aid in a thorough evaluation of the respiratory system by offering a detailed image of the lungs and surrounding structures.

By excluding other respiratory disorders that might exhibit symptoms similar to asthma, the combination of these diagnostic procedures enables medical professionals to make a precise and certain diagnosis of asthma. To start the right treatment plans and maximize asthma management, this accuracy is essential.

Evaluation of Severity and Categorization

Upon diagnosis, determining the severity of the condition and assigning it to a suitable category is crucial to creating a customized treatment regimen. The frequency and severity of symptoms as well as measurements of lung function from spirometry are used to estimate the severity of asthma.

Four frequent categories are used to classify asthma severity: mild persistent, moderate persistent, severe persistent, and intermittent. While chronic asthma categories show growing severity and frequency of symptoms, intermittent asthma is defined by rare and short episodes of symptoms. Healthcare professionals can use this classification system as a guide to select the best and most efficient drugs for managing asthma.

Spirometry, in particular, a lung function test, is essential for determining the severity of asthma. The findings aid in determining the extent of airflow restriction and direct medical professionals in choosing the best course of action. To provide the best possible control of asthma, treatment programs must be adjusted regularly based on lung function monitoring.

When evaluating severity, the effect of asthma on everyday activities and quality of life is taken into account in addition to clinical symptoms. More severe asthmatic patients could find it difficult to carry out their everyday activities and might need more intensive care to improve symptom control.

To sum up, classification and severity assessment are essential parts of managing asthma. Healthcare professionals can create individualized treatment regimens that cater to each patient's unique needs and improve overall well-being and symptom control by appropriately classifying the severity of asthma. Long-term asthma management requires routine monitoring and treatment plan modifications based on the patient's changing demands.

CHAPTER FOUR

COLLABORATING WITH MEDICAL PROFESSIONALS
Developing a Solid Patient-Doctor Bond

Building a strong rapport between the patient and the physician is essential to managing asthma effectively. The basis for effective cooperation between medical experts and patients suffering from this persistent respiratory ailment is this relationship. Encouragement of open communication is essential to developing this relationship. It is important for patients to feel at ease discussing their symptoms, experiences, and worries with their medical professionals. Doctors should, in turn, actively listen to their patients, validating their viewpoints and making sure the patient feels heard and understood.

An essential component of this relationship is trust. Patients with asthma must trust their healthcare providers to support them through the ups and downs of their disease, as managing the condition frequently involves a long-term commitment. However, doctors also need to have faith that their patients will follow their prescribed course of action and promptly report any changes or difficulties. Because of their shared trust, the parties form a cooperative collaboration that maximizes asthma control.

Additionally, fostering a solid patient-doctor connection requires education. Healthcare providers should empower people with asthma by educating them thoroughly about the disease, available treatments, and techniques for self-management. In addition to improving the patient's comprehension, this instruction promotes a feeling of shared accountability for the management of asthma.

In conclusion, open communication, reciprocal trust, and patient education are the cornerstones of a solid patient-doctor relationship in asthma care. By fostering a friendly atmosphere that encourages people to take an active role in their care, this foundation helps people manage their asthma more successfully.

Experts' Function in Asthma Management

Because asthma is a complicated and unpredictable illness, patients typically need specialized treatment to guarantee the best possible management and quality of life. Experts in their fields, such as pulmonologists and allergists, are vital to the all-encompassing management of asthma. Beyond basic primary care, these medical professionals offer a depth of knowledge and expertise.

As specialists in respiratory disorders, pulmonologists are well-versed in the complexities of asthma. To precisely determine the severity and origin of the ailment, they are prepared to carry out comprehensive diagnostic evaluations, which may include pulmonary function tests.

Because of this particular understanding, treatment programs can be customized to meet the unique requirements and difficulties faced by each patient.

With their emphasis on allergens and immune system reactions, allergists play a vital role in the treatment of asthma, particularly in cases when a patient's health is severely influenced by allergic triggers. Reducing the likelihood of exacerbations and managing these triggers can help manage the symptoms of asthma.

For comprehensive asthma care, primary care doctors and specialists must work together. Experts support the primary care team in making decisions based on the most recent findings and developments in asthma care. They also offer advice on advanced treatment options and insights into new medicines.

Fundamentally, the job of specialists in the treatment of asthma is to bring specific knowledge and expertise to the table, guaranteeing that patients receive the best possible care that is customized to the particulars of their illness.

Effective Communication with Your Medical Staff

One of the most important factors in the successful management of asthma is effective communication among the healthcare team. To offer complete treatment for patients with asthma, the team usually consists of primary care doctors, specialists, nurses, respiratory therapists, and other medical professionals. To guarantee that every facet of the patient's health is taken into account and treated, team members must communicate clearly and promptly with one another.

The exchange of thorough patient data is a crucial component of good communication. To make choices and deliver coordinated care, every member of the healthcare team should have access to pertinent medical information, test findings, and treatment plans. The healthcare team's efficiency is increased by the smooth sharing of information made possible by electronic health records and communication systems.

Frequent team meetings and case discussions create a collaborative environment that facilitates good communication. Through these forums, team members can discuss difficult situations, exchange thoughts, and work together to solve problems to improve patient outcomes. Furthermore, having open channels of communication guarantees that any modifications to the patient's condition or treatment plan are promptly shared with all members of the team, thereby avoiding gaps in care.

Engaging patients is another essential component of good communication. It is essential to support people with asthma in taking an active role in their care and to communicate pertinent details regarding their symptoms, triggers, and treatment compliance. Using a patient-centered approach improves diagnosis accuracy and makes customized care plans easier to implement.

In summary, thorough and well-coordinated therapy for asthma depends on the healthcare team's ability to communicate effectively with one another. The team may work together to address the various facets of asthma care by exchanging information, having cooperative talks, and encouraging patient participation. This will ultimately improve patient outcomes.

CHAPTER FIVE

PHARMACEUTICALS FOR ASTHMA
An Overview of Drugs for Asthma:

Wheezing, shortness of breath, pressure in the chest, and coughing are some of the symptoms associated with asthma, a long-term respiratory disease. Effective asthma management frequently entails a mix of environmental adjustments, lifestyle adjustments, and—most importantly—pharmaceuticals. People must comprehend the many kinds of asthma drugs to take charge of their symptoms and live a more satisfying life.

Asthma drugs fall into two basic categories: those intended for long-term control and those intended for rapid relief, or rescue. By treating the underlying inflammation in the airways, long-acting beta-agonists, leukotriene modifiers, and inhaled corticosteroids work to prevent the symptoms of asthma. Usually, regular use of these drugs is necessary to ensure steady control.

On the other hand, by relaxing the muscles around the airways, quick-relief drugs, such as short-acting beta-agonists, offer quick relief from acute asthma symptoms. By acting as bronchodilators, these drugs rapidly widen the airways, easing symptoms including dyspnea and wheezing. As needed, quick-relief drugs are used to treat acute asthma episodes or worsening symptoms.

Combination inhalers provide a complete strategy for managing asthma by targeting both inflammation and bronchoconstriction. They contain both long-acting bronchodilators and corticosteroids. Those with moderate to severe asthma are frequently prescribed these combo medicines.

Asthma patients must collaborate closely with their medical professionals to identify the best pharmacological plan for their requirements. To guarantee the best possible control of asthma, regular monitoring, and modifications to the treatment plan can be required.

Long-term care also requires a grasp of the need to keep follow-up appointments and take prescribed drugs as directed.

In conclusion, asthma drugs are essential for symptom management, averting flare-ups, and enhancing the general quality of life for those who have the condition. A customized strategy that takes into account the unique features of every patient's asthma is essential for effective treatment.

Nebulizers and inhalers: Correct Use Procedures

Nebulizers and inhalers are essential tools for administering asthma drugs directly to the lungs, resulting in both immediate and long-term symptom relief. To guarantee the efficacy of these devices and maximize the advantages of asthma drugs, proper usage procedures are essential.

Metered-dose inhalers (MDIs) are inhalers that provide medication in a precisely measured spray form. To guarantee that the drug reaches the lungs, the proper inhaler technique combines the inhaler's activation with a slow, deep inhale. Spacers are attachments for the inhaler that slow down the spray to improve medicine administration by facilitating effective inhalation.

Another kind of inhaler that gives medication in a powdered form is called a dry powder inhaler (DPI). A sharp, forceful inhale is necessary for proper dosage to distribute the medication evenly throughout the lungs. DPIs don't need you to press a canister and inhale at the same time as MDIs do.

In contrast, nebulizers turn liquid medication into a tiny mist that may be inhaled through a mouthpiece or mask. This technique is especially helpful for people who would have trouble using inhalers, like small toddlers or people experiencing acute respiratory distress. Nebulizers are a good option for people who have trouble breathing quickly enough to use inhalers since they give medication slowly and continuously.

For those with asthma, learning the right way to use a nebulizer and inhaler is essential to getting the most out of their medication. Healthcare professionals are essential in helping patients feel confident in their abilities to utilize these devices by demonstrating proper usage and offering continuing assistance.

In the end, becoming proficient with inhaler and nebulizer techniques gives asthmatics the ability to take charge of their care, proactively manage symptoms, and enhance their general respiratory health.

Comprehending Adverse Effects and Overseeing Drug Schedules:

Even though asthma drugs are necessary for controlling symptoms and averting exacerbations, it's critical to recognize that they could have adverse consequences. Important components of asthma management include being aware of these side effects and putting systems in place to efficiently manage prescription regimens.

Increased heart rate, hoarseness, oral thrush (a fungal infection in the mouth), and throat discomfort are common adverse effects of asthma drugs. One of the mainstays of long-term asthma treatment, inhaled corticosteroids, can also have systemic side effects, especially if taken for long periods and in high doses. Healthcare professionals collaborate closely with patients to properly monitor and manage these side effects, making necessary adjustments to prescription regimens to minimize unpleasant responses while maintaining symptom control.

For people with asthma, it's critical to schedule routine follow-up visits with medical professionals to talk about any new side effects and address any concerns. Good communication makes it possible to make timely changes to prescription schedules, which guarantees that the selected course of action is both efficient and well-tolerated.

Successful management of asthma requires not only an understanding of and ability to control side effects but also strict adherence to prescribed medication regimens. Together with patients, healthcare professionals develop individualized strategies that take into account each person's preferences, lifestyle, and asthma severity. Key components of an effective medication management plan include creating a regimen for administering medications, integrating them into everyday activities, and resolving any issues with adherence.

Moreover, knowledge about the identification and management of exacerbating symptoms or asthma episodes is beneficial for those who suffer from asthma. A thorough action plan that was created in conjunction with medical professionals instructs patients on when to change their medication, get help, or take rescue drugs.

In summary, proactive medication management and awareness of the possible adverse effects of asthma drugs are essential elements of good asthma care. Individuals diagnosed with asthma can effectively manage their treatment plans, attain optimal control over their symptoms, and experience an enhanced quality of life by maintaining continuous communication with healthcare providers and adhering to their prescribed regimens.

CHAPTER SIX

MANAGEMENT OF ENVIRONMENT AND LIFESTYLE
The Value of a Healthful Lifestyle in the Management of Asthma

Sustaining a healthy lifestyle is crucial for those who want to manage their asthma symptoms. If left untreated, asthma, a chronic respiratory disease marked by inflammation and airway constriction, can have a major negative influence on everyday activities. Changing to a healthier way of living can significantly reduce the frequency and intensity of asthma attacks. Maintaining a healthy weight, getting enough sleep, and engaging in regular physical activity all improve general well-being by strengthening the body's resistance to asthma triggers and lowering the risk of exacerbations.

In particular, exercise has a major role in enhancing cardiovascular and pulmonary health. Walking, swimming, and cycling are examples of exercises that assist in maintaining a healthy weight, which is important for managing asthma, in addition to strengthening respiratory muscles. Nonetheless, people with asthma must pick their activities wisely, taking into account their unique triggers. Additionally, a healthy diet high in foods high in antioxidants and anti-inflammatory properties can benefit respiratory health. Fruits, vegetables, and omega-3 fatty acids are examples of foods that have anti-inflammatory qualities and may lessen the severity of asthma symptoms.

The function of stress management in asthma control is equally significant. Stress can worsen symptoms and set off asthma attacks. Using stress-reduction methods such as yoga, meditation, and deep breathing can significantly improve general well-being. In addition, a healthy lifestyle for those with asthma includes going to frequent checkups with the doctor, taking prescribed drugs, and keeping up to date on health-related issues.

In summary, adopting a healthy lifestyle that includes constant medical treatment, frequent exercise, a balanced diet, and stress management is a key component of a holistic approach to asthma control. By empowering people to take control of their health, these techniques help people manage their asthma more proactively and live better overall.

Recognizing and Steering Clear of Asthma Triggers

One of the most important things in managing asthma is to recognize and stay away from anything that can cause respiratory distress. Each person has different asthma triggers, and understanding these triggers is crucial to managing the condition effectively. Allergens including mold, dust mites, pollen, and pet dander, as well as irritants like air pollution, tobacco smoke, and strong odors, are common triggers. Identifying one's unique triggers is essential to creating a customized asthma management strategy.

Identification of triggers can be aided by routine monitoring of environmental elements. Maintaining an extensive asthma journal that documents symptoms in connection with events, places, and exposures might yield important information. Furthermore, having an allergy test might assist in identifying particular allergens that might be causing symptoms of asthma.

The next stage is to put procedures in place to prevent or reduce exposure after triggers have been identified. For instance, installing enough ventilation can prevent mold formation, and employing air purifiers in the house can assist in lowering indoor air pollution. Establishing a "trigger-free" area in the bedroom that includes hypoallergenic bedding and a smoking ban can greatly enhance sleep and lessen symptoms of nocturnal asthma attacks.

A key element of trigger avoidance is education. People who suffer from asthma should be made aware of possible triggers and the appropriate safety measures to take. This involves knowing when to seek medical attention and how to use inhalers or other prescribed medications appropriately. People can greatly lower the frequency and intensity of asthma attacks, which improves overall asthma control and quality of life, by proactively identifying and avoiding triggers.

Creating a Home Environment That Is Asthma-Friendly

The home environment is critical to managing asthma and making a home asthma-friendly is essential for those who want to overcome their asthma with professional assistance. People spend a large amount of time at home, and respiratory health is directly impacted by the air quality in this setting. Taking proactive measures to reduce allergens and asthma triggers at home can help enhance general well-being.

Good allergen control is essential to making a house asthma-friendly. Common indoor allergens including mold, dust mites, pet dander, and pollen can worsen asthma symptoms. Frequent cleaning procedures can help lessen exposure to these triggers. These procedures include using a HEPA filter while vacuuming, washing bedding in hot water, and utilizing mattress and pillow covers that are allergen-proof. Further improving the quality of the air in the house is the prevention of mold formation through the maintenance of ideal humidity levels.

Taking action against indoor air pollution is another essential component. Indoor air quality can be greatly enhanced by routinely opening windows, employing exhaust fans, and abstaining from tobacco smoke. A healthier atmosphere can also be achieved by avoiding the use of air fresheners and scented candles and by using non-toxic cleaning supplies.

From a design perspective, designating a specific "clean air" area in the house, like the bedroom, might offer people a haven away from possible triggers. Using flooring options that are easy to clean, such as tile or hardwood, can help minimize the buildup of allergies.

Upholding an asthma-friendly environment in the home requires constant communication and education among family members. Family members should be informed about the person's asthma triggers and should encourage them to make the required lifestyle adjustments. Mold prevention and a healthy home environment depend on routine maintenance of heating and cooling systems and timely repair of any water leaks or damage.

To sum up, a coordinated effort to establish an asthma-friendly home environment entails a mix of allergy management, better air quality, and efficient communication within the family. By taking these steps, people who have asthma can greatly lessen the influence of outside variables on their respiratory health, making their living environment more comfortable and under control.

[47]

CHAPTER SEVEN

NUTRITION AND ASTHMA
The Role of Nutrition in Asthma Management

When it comes to treating asthma, a chronic respiratory disease marked by inflammation and airway narrowing, nutrition is crucial. Although prescription drugs are necessary to manage symptoms, a healthy, well-balanced diet can support conventional asthma treatment methods. A diet high in vitamins, minerals, and antioxidants promotes general respiratory health by lowering inflammation and bolstering the immune system.

The management of inflammation is a critical component of diet in the treatment of asthma. Eating foods strong in omega-3 fatty acids, such as flaxseeds, walnuts, and fatty fish, can help reduce inflammation in the airways. Furthermore, fruits and vegetables—especially those high in quercetin and vitamin C—have anti-inflammatory qualities that can help those who suffer from asthma. These nutrients might help stop chemicals from being released, which would otherwise constrict airways and exacerbate asthma symptoms.

Moreover, asthma management depends on keeping a healthy weight. Asthma is associated with obesity, and those who are overweight may have worsening symptoms. Regular exercise and a nutrient-dense, well-balanced diet will help control weight, which will ease the strain on the respiratory system and improve lung function overall.

People who suffer from asthma should be aware of possible trigger foods. While each person's relationship to certain foods and asthma triggers may be unique, dairy products, sulfites, and certain dietary additives are frequently implicated. A customized asthma treatment plan may include identifying and avoiding trigger foods.

In summary, diet plays a crucial role in managing asthma and has an impact that goes beyond just giving us food. For those who have asthma, a well-thought-out anti-inflammatory diet full of vital nutrients can make a big difference in lowering inflammation, boosting immunity, and helping with weight management.

Foods That Could Help Reduce the Symptoms of Asthma

Some meals have been found to have the ability to improve lung health and reduce symptoms of asthma. These items can be added to a balanced diet to help manage asthma in addition to the conventional methods. Antioxidant-rich foods are one type of food that has drawn attention in this context.

Foods high in antioxidants, such as citrus fruits, berries, and dark leafy greens, are essential in scavenging free radicals that cause inflammation in the respiratory system. Strong antioxidants include vitamins A, C, and E, and minerals like selenium can be found in a variety of fruits and vegetables. By shielding the respiratory system from oxidative stress, these nutrients may lessen the intensity and frequency of asthma attacks.

Omega-3 fatty acids are abundant in fatty fish, including mackerel and salmon, and are well-known for their anti-inflammatory qualities. Consuming these fish could help people with asthma feel better by reducing the inflammatory response in their airways. Omega-3 fatty acids can also be found in nuts and seeds, especially walnuts and flaxseeds, which can be beneficial additions to a diet that is asthma-friendly.

Foods high in probiotics, such as yogurt and vegetables that have undergone fermentation, support a balanced gut microbiota. Recent studies point to a connection between respiratory disorders, such as asthma, and gastrointestinal health. Probiotics may influence the degree of asthma symptoms by regulating immune responses and lowering inflammation.

In conclusion, adding probiotics, omega-3 fatty acids, and foods high in antioxidants to the diet can help prevent asthma symptoms. Although these meals shouldn't take the place of prescription drugs, they can be beneficial supplements to a comprehensive asthma management program, improving respiratory health and general well-being.

Dietary Strategies to Prevent Asthma

Adopting dietary habits that promote respiratory health and reduce potential triggers is part of preventing asthma. A proactive dietary strategy can help manage symptoms in individuals who have already been diagnosed with asthma and lower the chance of getting the condition. Keeping a well-balanced diet that delivers important nutrients to promote overall health is a fundamental part of asthma prevention.

Consuming a diet high in fruits and vegetables guarantees that one is getting enough vitamins, minerals, and antioxidants—all of which are essential for immune system support and lung function. These nutrient-dense foods contribute to a strong respiratory system, potentially reducing the susceptibility to asthma-related disorders.

Stressing the need for a diet rich in whole grains, healthy fats, and a range of lean meats is also crucial for general well-being. Fish, poultry, and legumes are good sources of lean protein and include important amino acids needed for proper muscular function, especially in the respiratory muscles. In addition to supporting general cardiovascular health and maintaining energy levels, whole grains and healthy fats can indirectly improve respiratory function.

Another essential component of dietary strategies for preventing asthma is staying hydrated. Maintaining proper hydration facilitates the production of mucus at its best and keeps airways wet, which may lessen the likelihood of irritation and inflammation. It's crucial to drink enough water while you're in dry or low-humidity conditions because these conditions might exacerbate respiratory pain.

One of the most important dietary strategies for preventing asthma attacks is avoiding possible trigger foods. While each person may have different trigger foods, dairy products, processed foods, and foods with artificial chemicals are frequently identified as offenders. Finding and removing trigger items from the diet can help lower the chance of developing asthma or having symptoms worsen.

In conclusion, a proactive strategy for preventing asthma is to adopt dietary practices that emphasize nutrient-dense foods, staying hydrated, and avoiding trigger foods. A balanced, conscientious diet can greatly improve respiratory health and lower the risk of asthma-related problems, although genetics and environmental factors also matter.

CHAPTER EIGHT

ACTIVITY LEVELS AND ASTHMA
Advantages of Exercise for People with Asthma:

Contrary to the common belief that exercise aggravates asthma, regular physical activity provides several benefits for those who suffer from the condition. An organized exercise program helps improve cardiovascular health and lung function, which are important factors for asthma sufferers. Increased respiratory muscle endurance and strength is one main benefit. Regular exercise helps the respiratory muscles become more effective, which facilitates better breathing and lessens the sensation of being out of breath.

Exercise also helps with weight management, which is important for managing asthma. Keeping a healthy weight lessens the burden on the respiratory system and lowers the risk of asthma episodes. Furthermore, exercise strengthens the immune system and lowers the chance of respiratory infections, which can exacerbate asthma symptoms. Improved cardiovascular fitness is another important advantage since it increases the body's effectiveness in utilizing oxygen, which lessens the strain on the respiratory system when engaging in physical activity.

Additionally, regular exercise has a favorable effect on mental health, which is linked to managing asthma. Endorphins are released when we exercise, which elevates our mood and lowers our stress levels. Exercise helps manage stress, which can be a cause of asthma exacerbations, and improves overall asthma control.

In conclusion, exercise has advantages for asthmatics that go beyond simple physical healing. An all-encompassing approach to asthma therapy benefits from the beneficial effects on respiratory muscles, weight management, immunological function, cardiovascular fitness, and mental well-being.

Selecting Appropriate Exercises:

For people with asthma, choosing the right physical activities is essential to maximizing the health benefits of exercise and reducing the chance of exacerbating symptoms. Activities that range from mild to moderate in intensity are usually well-tolerated and advised. Walking, swimming, and cycling are great examples of aerobic exercises because they improve cardiovascular fitness without overtaxing the respiratory system.

Choosing exercises that grow gradually is crucial since this allows the body to gradually adjust to higher levels of effort. For asthma sufferers, warm-up and cool-down phases are essential parts of every workout regimen. These lessen the chance of asthma symptoms by helping the body get ready for physical exercise and preventing abrupt increases in breathing and heart rate.

Activity selection should be based on personal interests and health considerations. Due to its relaxing effects, some people may find group activities like yoga or Tai Chi more suited, while others may find solitary hobbies like jogging more appropriate. It's critical to pay attention to one's body and recognize one's boundaries because exerting too much energy can exacerbate asthma attacks.

In summary, the best physical activities for people with asthma are those that balance increasing fitness with reducing the chance of exacerbating symptoms. A customized strategy that takes into account each person's interests and health situation guarantees a fun and long-lasting workout regimen.

Exercise Safety and Asthma Management:

Exercise is good for people with asthma, but there are some things you should know to keep yourself safe and avoid aggravating your condition. People should speak with their healthcare professionals to evaluate their asthma management and obtain customized recommendations before beginning any fitness program. Identifying and sharing one's asthma triggers with the medical team is essential to creating a customized exercise program that reduces risks.

When exercising, it is imperative to pay attention to the surrounding surroundings. Some asthmatics may have bronchoconstriction when exercising in cold or dry air. One way to reduce this danger is to wear a scarf or mask to warm and humidify the air before inhaling. It's crucial to monitor the quality of the air, particularly when engaging in outdoor activities, as low air quality might worsen respiratory problems.

A well-considered asthma action strategy is essential. This strategy ought to outline instructions for modifying medicine, seeing early warning indications of deteriorating symptoms, and understanding when to consult a doctor. Having a rescue inhaler on hand and making sure it's accessible during physical activity is essential for quick response in the event of an asthma attack.

In conclusion, a well-defined action plan, medical advice, and environmental awareness are all important components of asthma safety precautions. People with asthma can safely participate in physical activity and benefit from it while reducing the danger to their respiratory health if they take these precautions.

CHAPITRE NINE

COMPLEMENTARY METHODS AND ALTERNATIVE THERAPIES
Synopsis of Complementary Medicine

Alternative therapies, which emphasize holistic methods that go beyond traditional medical treatments, provide a wide range of possibilities for managing asthma.

Taking into account the connection between the mind and body, these treatments seek to treat the underlying reasons for asthma symptoms. A well-known alternative treatment is acupuncture, which stimulates energy flow by inserting tiny needles into predetermined body locations.

By encouraging relaxation and lowering inflammation, acupuncture has demonstrated promise in easing the symptoms of asthma and enhancing lung function.

Another complementary therapy that is becoming more well-known for its beneficial effects on asthma control is yoga. Yoga's physical postures, breathing techniques, and meditation combine to strengthen respiratory muscles, expand lung capacity, and improve general well-being. Yoga promotes conscious breathing, which is advantageous for those who have asthma since it helps control breathing patterns and lowers stress, which is a common cause of asthma episodes.

An essential part of alternative asthma treatments is breathing exercises like pursed-lip breathing and the Buteyko method. These methods emphasize controlled, slow breathing patterns to retrain the respiratory system. Specifically, the Buteyko approach seeks to restore breathing and lessen hyperventilation, which in turn lessens asthma symptoms. Exhaling through pursed lips helps keep airways open and enhances ventilation-perfusion matching, which lessens breathing effort for asthmatic patients.

Yoga, Acupuncture, and Breathing Methods

One of the main non-pharmacological treatments for asthma is acupuncture, which involves putting tiny needles into certain body locations to increase energy flow and bring the body back into equilibrium. According to research, acupuncture may help asthma by lowering inflammation and altering the immune system.

Acupuncturists try to relieve symptoms including tightness in the chest, wheezing, and shortness of breath by focusing on particular acupuncture sites. Furthermore, acupuncture sessions frequently encourage relaxation, which may lessen asthma triggers connected to stress.

Yoga provides a holistic approach to asthma care with a focus on physical postures, breath control, and meditation. Yoga's physical component strengthens the muscles of the respiratory system and enhances lung function. Certain yoga positions, like those that emphasize opening up the chest, can improve lung capacity. In the meantime, pranayama, or breath control, trains people to intentionally manage their breathing. This feature of yoga is especially helpful for people who have asthma because it encourages breath awareness and helps reduce hyperventilation, which is a typical cause of asthma attacks.

Breathing exercises are essential to alternative asthma treatment plans. Shallow breathing exercises are part of the Buteyko method, which was created to treat chronic hyperventilation and restore normal respiratory patterns.

The goal of this technique is to lessen the dependence on rapid, shallow breathing, which can make asthma symptoms worse. Another method is pursed-lip breathing, which is exhaling via pursed lips to provide resistance that prolongs airway opening. Through the treatment of the underlying patterns of disordered breathing, these treatments not only enhance respiratory efficiency but also aid in the overall management of asthma symptoms.

Combining Complementary Methods with Traditional Therapy

A comprehensive approach to improving overall care and symptom management for asthma patients is the integration of complementary therapies with traditional asthma treatment. While anti-inflammatory drugs and bronchodilators, which are examples of conventional treatments, concentrate on symptom relief and averting exacerbations, complementary therapies address the larger picture of health, which includes psychological and emotional variables that might affect asthma.

A major advantage of using complementary methods is that there may be less need for prescription drugs and the negative effects that go along with them. People with asthma may be able to better control their condition by utilizing methods like acupuncture, yoga, and breathing exercises. This would enable them to better manage their medication under the supervision of medical professionals. Additionally, by addressing unique requirements and preferences, complementary treatments help to create a more patient-centered approach to asthma therapy.

Complementary treatments address the psychological components of asthma because they are holistic. Asthma symptoms can be exacerbated by worry and stress, and complementary therapies offer strategies for relaxation and stress management.

When combined with complementary techniques, mindfulness practices enable people to take charge of their mental health and may even lessen the frequency and intensity of asthma attacks.

In summary, a comprehensive strategy for treating this long-term respiratory ailment is provided by combining complementary and alternative therapies with traditional asthma medication. A variety of choices are available for people with asthma to investigate in conjunction with healthcare providers, ranging from the traditional Chinese medicine of acupuncture to the all-encompassing advantages of yoga and focused breathing techniques.

This combined strategy promotes a more thorough and individualized approach to asthma management by addressing not only the physical components of asthma but also the interconnections between mental and emotional well-being.

CHAPTER TEN

HANDLING ASTHMA ACROSS AGE GROUPS
Children's Asthma: Special Considerations

Childhood asthma is a chronic respiratory disease that presents special difficulties. Children's asthma needs to be managed differently because of their unique behavioral patterns and developing respiratory systems.

The challenge of diagnosing asthma in very young children, which frequently depends on clinical symptoms and family history, is an important factor to take into account. The treatment of asthma in children places a strong emphasis on individualized care regimens that are based on the child's age, the severity of their symptoms, and their triggers.

It's critical to identify and deal with triggers in children. Exposure to environmental irritants, allergies, and respiratory infections are common factors. Pediatricians and allergists frequently work together to pinpoint certain triggers and create avoidance plans. Furthermore, it might be difficult for patients to follow their drug regimen, which calls for age-appropriate delivery methods and vigilant parental supervision. Nebulizers and inhalers with spacers are frequently employed to guarantee efficient drug delivery.

One of the most important aspects of managing childhood asthma is education. Parents and other caregivers must be knowledgeable about the illness, available treatments, and emergency protocols. Essential tools for managing asthma are action plans, which include step-by-step directions for everyday management and what to do in the event of an exacerbation. It is crucial to schedule routine check-ups with medical professionals to assess lung function, modify medication regimens, and handle any new issues.

Furthermore, it's critical to encourage open communication with the child. Promoting age-appropriate dialogues on the emotions and symptoms of asthma increases awareness and gives kids the confidence to actively participate in their treatment. Asthma education should be extended to childcare facilities and schools to provide a welcoming environment that meets the needs of the kids.

Teens and Adolescents with Asthma

Managing asthma becomes entwined with the difficulties of independence, peer pressure, and changing self-identity during the transitional period of adolescence. Teens and adolescents may be more likely to mishandle their medical conditions, underestimate how serious their asthma is, or give in to peer pressure that can make asthma triggers like smoking or allergen exposure worse.

When working with this age group, healthcare providers need to take a compassionate stance, recognizing their increasing independence and stressing the value of ongoing asthma treatment. It's critical to modify treatment regimens to fit the tastes and lifestyles of adolescents. This could entail talking about how lifestyle decisions affect asthma and looking into inhaler solutions that work well with their everyday schedules.

Adolescent asthma management is significantly influenced by psychosocial variables as well. Improving the management of stressors, anxiety, and body image issues can help improve asthma control. Teenage asthma education programs might include interactive components to get them involved in their care, including peer support groups or online tools.

Furthermore, the shift from pediatric to adult care must be gradual and well-planned. Adolescents require assistance in managing their health, comprehending insurance, and navigating the adult healthcare system. To guarantee a seamless transition and ongoing asthma control, this phase calls for cooperation between parents, healthcare professionals, and the teenagers themselves.

Adult and Senior Asthma Management

The dynamics of managing asthma continue to change as people become older. When it comes to adults, the focus switches to managing chronic symptoms effectively and avoiding flare-ups. Healthcare professionals create thorough asthma action plans with adult patients that include rescue inhalers, daily medicines, and lifestyle changes.

Comorbid conditions like osteoporosis or cardiovascular disease might make controlling asthma more difficult for seniors. When prescribing asthma drugs, any drug interactions and contraindications need to be carefully considered. The choice of treatment modalities may also be influenced by age-related changes in immune response and lung capacity, with inhalers and nebulizers frequently being favored over oral drugs.

In the management of adult and senior asthma, environmental factors become more important. An essential part of care is recognizing and addressing triggers at home and work. The main goal should be quitting smoking, if it is applicable since tobacco smoke aggravates asthma symptoms and reduces the efficacy of treatment.

For adults and older people, it is crucial to regularly assess lung function using spirometry and other diagnostic testing. This enables medical professionals to quickly modify treatment regimens, guaranteeing the best possible control of asthma. Throughout adulthood, patient education is ongoing, with a focus on self-management strategies and knowledge of warning signals that could point to declining respiratory function.

In conclusion, treating asthma in varying age groups necessitates a sophisticated and customized strategy. Comprehensive and efficient asthma care is ensured by taking into account the particular factors of every period of life, from childhood through adolescence to adulthood and older years.

CHAPTER ELEVEN

ASTHMA CARE'S FUTURE TRENDS AND INNOVATIONS
New Media and the Handling of Asthma:

With the introduction of new technologies, the field of asthma care is changing quickly and ushering in a new era of effective and individualized therapy. The emergence of digital health solutions, such as wearable technology, and smartphone apps, that are intended to track and treat asthma symptoms in real time is one noteworthy development. With the use of these devices, people may monitor their respiratory health and gain valuable insights into trends and triggers that might be essential for managing their asthma.

With its sensors and Bluetooth connectivity, smart inhalers are a revolutionary advancement in the treatment of asthma. These devices enable patients and healthcare professionals to monitor adherence and spot any problems by not only delivering medication but also recording usage data. More informed decisions may be made thanks to this data-driven approach, which enables treatment regimens to be modified in response to individual reactions and trends.

Another game-changing technological advancement that is having an impact on asthma care is artificial intelligence (AI). Large datasets can be analyzed by machine learning algorithms, which can then be used to find relationships between treatment outcomes, genetics, and environmental factors. This makes it possible to identify asthma phenotypes with greater accuracy, opening the door to individualized treatment plans. Predictive models driven by artificial intelligence (AI) can forecast asthma flare-ups, facilitating early management and lessening the demand for emergency medical services.

The use of telemedicine has grown, particularly when it comes to managing asthma. Patients can easily communicate with medical professionals, discuss symptoms, and get advice on therapy modifications through virtual consultations. This method improves accessibility, especially for people who live in distant places or have limited mobility.

In conclusion, new technology in asthma treatment is changing the established models of care. Artificial intelligence, smart inhalers, and digital health tools are just a few examples of the advancements that give patients and healthcare professionals useful information that may be used to manage asthma more effectively and individually.

Research Developments and Hopeful Therapies:

Advances in science are changing the way that asthma is treated, providing fresh hope and opportunities for better results. Understanding asthma heterogeneity and distinguishing between different phenotypes is one exciting field of research. This personalized approach to the categorization of asthma moves beyond the traditional one-size-fits-all paradigm by enabling targeted therapies based on individual patient profiles.

In the treatment of severe asthma, biological treatments, or biologics, have become a game-changer. These drugs, which are frequently monoclonal antibodies, target particular immune system pathways that cause allergic reactions. Biologics efficiently regulate symptoms in individuals who do not react well to conventional medicines by precisely modifying immune activity. For people with severe, refractory asthma in particular, this is a breakthrough.

Gene therapy appears to be a promising avenue for treating asthma in the future. Comprehending the genetic foundations of asthma vulnerability enables the creation of focused treatments meant to alter or rectify malfunctioning genes. Gene therapy, which targets the underlying molecular causes of asthma, has the potential to completely transform asthma treatment, even if it is still in its early phases of research.

Additionally, new anti-inflammatory drugs are being researched to supplement current therapeutic approaches. Small molecule medications that target particular inflammatory pathways provide an alternative for individuals who do not respond well to existing treatments or who suffer side effects. These cutting-edge medications seek to improve asthma care by offering more thorough inflammation control.

In conclusion, continuing research is revealing previously undiscovered aspects of asthma and opening the door to novel therapies. The future of asthma management is promising, with personalized therapies based on phenotypes, gene therapy, biologics, and innovative anti-inflammatory medicines all on the horizon.

The Changing Face of Asthma Management

A comprehensive approach to asthma care that addresses the wider variables influencing lung health in addition to symptom management is bringing about a revolutionary change in the field. With an emphasis on lifestyle changes and self-management techniques, patient education and empowerment are fast taking center stage in the treatment of asthma.

The use of integrated care models is growing, encouraging cooperation between pulmonologists, allergists, primary care physicians, and respiratory therapists, among other medical specialists. Through the treatment of both the underlying causes of asthma exacerbations and the immediate symptoms, this multidisciplinary approach guarantees thorough and coordinated care. Shared decision-making is used to create patient-centric care plans that take into account each patient's preferences and objectives.

The importance of environmental factors in asthma treatment is becoming more well-acknowledged. This entails using home evaluations and treatments to identify and mitigate environmental triggers, such as pollution and allergies. The focus on environmental factors is extended to public health policies and urban planning, to develop communities that are hospitable to people with asthma and reduce exposure hazards.

In the ever-changing field of asthma care, community involvement, and support systems are vital. People with asthma can exchange experiences, coping techniques, and tactics on forums such as peer support groups and online communities. These networks lessen the social isolation that people with long-term illnesses may experience and foster a feeling of community.

Value-based care models are changing the way that healthcare is delivered by placing more emphasis on quality of life and results than on the quantity of services rendered. To reduce exacerbations and hospital stays, this translates into an emphasis on preventative measures; early intervention, and ongoing monitoring in the context of asthma management. The objective is to lessen the financial burden that comes with uncontrolled disease while also improving the general well-being of people who have asthma.

To sum up, the way asthma care is developing indicates a paradigm change in favor of proactive, patient-centered, holistic approaches. Through the implementation of integrated care models, community engagement, environmental influences mitigation, and value-based care, the healthcare system can more effectively improve the quality of life for asthmatic patients and lessen the burden of this chronic illness on society at large.

www.ingramcontent.com/pod-product-compliance
Lightning Source LLC
Chambersburg PA
CBHW050742260726
48661CB00001B/373